The Easiest Low Carb Diet Cookbook for Beginners

2021 EDITION

Contents

Instant Pot Low carb Corned Beef Brisket

No Bean Whole30 Keto Chili In The Instant Pot

Low carb Bacon Cheeseburger Soup – Instant Pot Recipe

Instant Pot Chicken Tikka Masala

Healthy Chicken Pot Pie Soup

BALSAMIC CHICKEN [INSTANT POT]

INSTANT POT SHRIMP WITH TOMATOES AND FETA | GREEK SHRIMP SAGANAKI

INSTANT POT ORANGE CHICKEN RECIPE

PUMPKIN CHICKEN CURRY (INSTANT POT)

INSTANT POT LAMB STEW

BBQ Instant Pot Whole Chicken

Instant Pot Cuban-style beef lettuce wraps

Instant Pot Whole Roasted Cauliflower With Chimichurri Sauce

Instant Pot Turmeric Tahini Chicken Soup

INSTANT POT STEAK FAJITAS RECIPE

No Noodle Lasagna

THAI GREEN CURRY RECIPE

Crazy Good Instant Pot Pork Carnitas

Instant Pot Mexican Stuffed Sweet Potatoes

LEMON CHICKEN SOUP (INSTANT POT)

Easy Instant Pot Ribs Recipe

INSTANT POT TACO SOUP

Instant Pot Summer Soup

INSTANT POT SALSA CHICKEN

INSTANT POT HUNGARIAN POT ROAST

INSTANT POT SOUTHWESTERN BEEF STEW

GREEN CHILE CHICKEN BURRITO BOWL

INSTANT POT SOUTHWESTERN POT ROAST

INSTANT POT BALSAMIC PORK ROAST

INSTANT POT CAULIFLOWER RICE GREEK CHICKEN BOWLS

SPICY SHREDDED CHICKEN LETTUCE WRAP TACOS

INTRODUCTION

A low-carb diet is a diet that restricts carbohydrates, such as those found in sugary foods, pasta and bread. It is high in protein, fat and healthy vegetables.

There are many different types of low-carb diets, and studies show that they can cause weight loss and improve health.

Instant Pot is a multi-cooker that can be used as an electric pressure cooker, slow cooker, steamer, yogurt maker, rice cooker, sauté/browning pan, and warming pot. In nutshell, Instant Pot does the job of seven kitchen tools or appliances.

Instant Pot is quite convenient and dependable. It can speed up your cooking by 2-6 times by consuming up to 70% less energy, and, above all, produce healthy and nutritious food in a consistent and convenient fashion.

In nutshell, if you are living in a fast-paced, green-conscious, and health-oriented life style, Instant Pot is definitely for you.

This is a detailed meal plan for a low-carb diet. It explains what to eat, what to avoid and includes a sample low-carb menu for one week, easy and quick delicious recipes for your pressure cooker.

LOW-CARB EATING — THE BASICS

Your food choices depend on a few things, including how healthy you are, how much you exercise and how much weight you have to lose.

Consider this meal plan as a general guideline, not something written in stone.

Eat: Meat, fish, eggs, vegetables, fruit, nuts, seeds, high-fat dairy, fats, healthy oils and maybe even some tubers and non-gluten grains.

Don't eat: Sugar, HFCS, wheat, seed oils, trans fats, "diet" and low-fat products and highly processed foods.

FOODS TO AVOID

You should avoid these six food groups and nutrients, in order of importance:

• Sugar: Soft drinks, fruit juices, agave, candy, ice cream and many other products that contain added sugar.

• Refined grains: Wheat, rice, barley and rye, as well as bread, cereal and pasta.

• Trans fats: Hydrogenated or partially hydrogenated oils.

• Diet and low-fat products: Many dairy products, cereals or crackers are fat-reduced, but contain added sugar.

• Highly processed foods: If it looks like it was made in a factory, don't eat it.

• Starchy vegetables: It's best to limit starchy vegetables in your diet if you're following a very low-carb diet.

You must read ingredient lists even on foods labelled as health foods.

LOW-CARB FOOD LIST — FOODS TO EAT

You should base your diet on these real, unprocessed, low-carb foods.

• Meat: Beef, lamb, pork, chicken and others; grass-fed is best.

• Fish: Salmon, trout, haddock and many others; wild-caught fish is best.

• Eggs: Omega-3-enriched or pastured eggs are best.

• Vegetables: Spinach, broccoli, cauliflower, carrots and many others.

• Fruits: Apples, oranges, pears, blueberries, strawberries.

• Nuts and seeds: Almonds, walnuts, sunflower seeds, etc.

• High-fat dairy: Cheese, butter, heavy cream, yogurt.

• Fats and oils: Coconut oil, butter, lard, olive oil and fish oil.

If you need to lose weight, be careful with cheese and nuts, as it's easy to overeat on them. Don't eat more than one piece of fruit per day.

FOODS TO MAYBE INCLUDE

If you're healthy, active and don't need to lose weight, you can afford to eat a few more carbs.

• Tubers: Potatoes, sweet potatoes and some others.

• Unrefined grains: Brown rice, oats, quinoa and many others.

• Legumes: Lentils, black beans, pinto beans, etc. (if you can tolerate them).

What's more, you can have the following in moderation, if you want:

• Dark chocolate: Choose organic brands with at least 70% of cocoa.

• Wine: Choose dry wines with no added sugar or carbs.

Dark chocolate is high in antioxidants and may provide health benefits if you eat it in moderation. However, be aware that both dark chocolate and alcohol will hinder your progress if you eat/drink too much.

• Beverages

• Coffee

• Tea

• Water

• Sugar-free carbonated beverages, like sparkling water.

A SAMPLE LOW-CARB MENU FOR ONE WEEK

This is a sample menu for one week on a low-carb diet plan.

It provides less than 50 grams of total carbs per day. However, if you're healthy and active you can eat slightly more carbs.

Monday

Breakfast: Omelet with various vegetables, fried in butter or coconut oil.

Lunch: Grass-fed yogurt with blueberries and a handful of almonds.

Dinner: Bunless cheeseburger, served with vegetables and salsa sauce.

Tuesday

Breakfast: Bacon and eggs.

Lunch: Leftover burgers and veggies from the previous night.

Dinner: Salmon with butter and vegetables.

Wednesday

Breakfast: Eggs and vegetables, fried in butter or coconut oil.

Lunch: Shrimp salad with some olive oil.

Dinner: Grilled chicken with vegetables.

Thursday

Breakfast: Omelet with various vegetables, fried in butter or coconut oil.

Lunch: Smoothie with coconut milk, berries, almonds and protein powder.

Dinner: Steak and veggies.

Friday

Breakfast: Bacon and eggs.

Lunch: Chicken salad with some olive oil.

Dinner: Pork chops with vegetables.

Saturday
Breakfast: Omelet with various veggies.

Lunch: Grass-fed yogurt with berries, coconut flakes and a handful of walnuts.

Dinner: Meatballs with vegetables.

Sunday
Breakfast: Bacon and eggs.

Lunch: Smoothie with coconut milk, a dash of heavy cream, chocolate-flavored protein powder and berries.

Dinner: Grilled chicken wings with some raw spinach on the side.

Include plenty of low-carb vegetables in your diet. If your goal is to remain under 50 grams of carbs per day, there is room for plenty of veggies and one fruit per day.

Again, if you're healthy, lean and active, you can add some tubers like potatoes and sweet potatoes, as well as some healthy grains like oats.

HEALTHY, LOW-CARB SNACKS

There is no health reason to eat more than three meals per day, but if you get hungry between meals, here are some healthy, easy-to-prepare, low-carb snacks that can fill you up:

- A piece of fruit

- Full-fat yogurt

- One or two hard-boiled eggs

- Baby carrots

- Leftovers from the previous night

- A handful of nuts

- Some cheese and meat

EATING AT RESTAURANTS

At most restaurants, it's fairly easy to make your meals low-carb friendly.

• Order a meat- or fish-based main dish.

• Drink plain water instead of sugary soda or fruit juice.

• Get extra vegetables instead of bread, potatoes or rice.

A SIMPLE LOW-CARB SHOPPING LIST

A good rule is to shop at the perimeter of the store, where the whole foods are more likely to be found.

Focusing on whole foods will make your diet a thousand times better than the standard Western diet.

Organic and grass-fed foods are also popular choices and often considered healthier, but they're typically more expensive.

Try to choose the least processed option that still fits into your price range.

• Meat (beef, lamb, pork, chicken, bacon)

• Fish (fatty fish like salmon is best)

• Eggs (choose omega-3 enriched or pastured eggs if you can)

• Butter

• Coconut oil

• Lard

• Olive oil

• Cheese

• Heavy cream

• Sour cream

• Yogurt (full-fat, unsweetened)

• Blueberries (fresh or frozen)

• Nuts

• Olives

• Fresh vegetables (greens, peppers, onions, etc.)

• Frozen vegetables (broccoli, carrots, various mixes)

• Condiments (sea salt, pepper, garlic, mustard, etc.)

Clear your pantry of all unhealthy temptations if you can, such as chips, candy, ice cream, sodas, juices, breads, cereals and baking ingredients like refined flour and sugar.

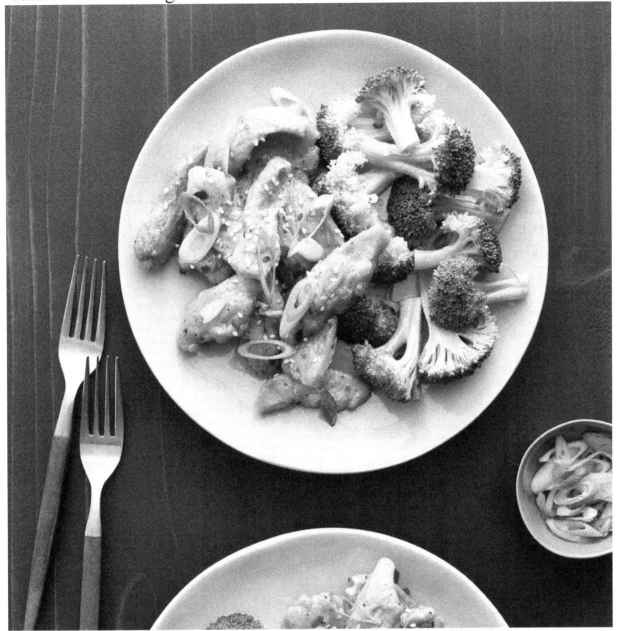

WHAT IS INSTANT POT?

Instant Pot is a multi-cooker that can be used as an electric pressure cooker, slow cooker, steamer, yogurt maker, rice cooker, sauté/browning pan, and warming pot. In nutshell, Instant Pot does the job of seven kitchen tools or appliances.

Instant Pot is quite convenient and dependable. It can speed up your cooking by 2-6 times by consuming up to 70% less energy, and, above all, produce healthy and nutritious food in a consistent and convenient fashion.

In nutshell, if you are living in a fast-paced, green-conscious, and health-oriented life style, Instant Pot is definitely for you.

WHY INSTANT POT?

The following five aspects summarize the benefits of Instant Pot:

1. Convenient

Instant Pot comes with 12 turn-key function keys to perform your most common cooking tasks and to save your cooking time up to 70%.

These common tasks includes:

- Congee/Porridge
- Sauté/Browning Soup
- Poultry
- Meat & Stew
- Rice
- Multigrain rice
- Beans & Chili
- Steaming
- Slow Cook
- Keep warm
- Yogurt

These keys are precisely and carefully designed to provide you consistent cooking results. Of course, it provides you manual setting as well in case you want to set up pressure keeping time for your own recipe.

These one-button operation keys are notable for the following features:

Intelligent Programming

These 12 keys are intelligently programmed after many experiments to achieve best results.

Let's take the "Rice" button as an example. While cooking rice, Instant Pot assess the amount of water and rice by calculating the pre-heating time. The duration of keeping the pressure is then calculated based on this measurement. Detailed attention is given in each of the stages of rice cooking, that is, soak, blanch, steam, and braise.

Each key can be further enhanced by varying the food taste in the range of normal, rare, and well-done.

Automatic Cooking

Instant Pot is an automated cooking process that time each cooking task and can keep the food warm even after cooking. Unlike traditional pressure cookers, you don't have to manually monitor the cooking time.

Delayed Cooking and Meal Planning

Instant Pot can delay your cooking for up to 24 hours that allows you to plan your meal well in advance. Most importantly, you don't have to spend time in the kitchen to watch the cooking operations.

2. - Cooking nutritious, healthy, and tasty meals

Pressure cooking in Instant Pot helps in cooking a meal, softening the food, and retaining vitamins/minerals. This is achieved by its micro-processor controlled cooking cycles that cook a meal in a consistent fashion.

Retain Flavor in Food

Cooking in Instant Pot is a fully sealed process. Hence, aroma and nutrients stay in the ingredients instead of being dispersed around the house. For example, the original juice of meat, fruits, or juice remains within the food.

Keep Minerals and Vitamins Intact

Steaming with Instant Pot does not require you to fill a large amount of water. It just needs enough water to keep the cooker filled with steam. Hence, the minerals and vitamins remain intact and do not dissolve away by water. This helps in avoiding food to get oxidized by air exposure at heat and that means broccoli, asparagus, and so on will retain their phytochemicals and bright green colors.

Tasty & Tender Meal

Instant Pot cooks bones and meat really tender. It separates the bone pork ribs from the meat after cooking and they become chewable and it preserves the necessary calcium and other minerals.

Under pressure cooking, the whole grain and bean based meals taste better than any of the traditional cooking methods.

3. - Clean & Pleasant

The traditional cooker has an image of a spitting, steaming monster that nosily rattles on the stove, which is no longer true with Instant Pot.

Instant Pot is extremely quite during the cooking time. The steam does not escape from the pot as Instant Pot is fully sealed. That means no more food smell in your kitchen and home, and flavors and aroma of your food remain intact.

Instant Pot is a perfect kitchen tool for summers as it cooks food without heating up the surroundings and saves your electricity consumption during heating and cooling of the kitchen.

Another amazing benefit of Instant pot is that it keeps your kitchen clean. You don't have to clean any splashes, spills, or spatters and no more boiled over foods. You can be rest assured that aroma of your food is trapped in the food and it will be released on when you open the lid.

4. - Energy Efficient

Instant Pot can save up to 70% of your electricity and thus makes it one of the greenest kitchen appliances. Thanks to the following features that make it a highly energy efficient cooking tool:

i. Firstly, it cooks rapidly under high-temperature and saves you up to 70% of the cooking time. Less cooking time equals to less energy consumed.

ii. Secondly, Instant Pot exterior comes with fully insulated two layers of air pockets between the exterior and the inner pot and, hence, energy is focused on cooking the food. This makes it more energy efficient than any of the traditional pressure cookers.

iii. Thirdly, Instant Pot maintains certain pressure level by heating only the inner pot. Thanks to its intelligent monitoring system, the heating is almost 40% off during a long hours cooking.

iv. Fourthly, Instant Pot consumes lesser water than normal cooking as it's fully sealed during cooking. This reduces the overall energy consumption in making the meal.

5. - Absolutely Dependable and Safe

Instant Pot comes with 10 level of safety protections:

1) Lid Close Detection

Instant Pot will not activate pressure cooking if the lid is missing or not closed properly. Only the sauté and keep-warm functions work with the open lid.

2) Leaky Lid Protection

A cooker cannot reach its preset pressure level if there is a leakage in the cooker lid. In this scenario, the food is also at risk of burning out. Instant Pot senses this by measuring the pre-heating time and if the pre-heating time is longer than the normal, Instant Pot switches itself to the Keep-warm mode to avoid the food to be burnt out.

3) Lid Lock under Pressure

Instant Pot lid will be locked if the cooker is still pressurized. This is to avoid accidental opening.

4) Anti-blockage Vent

During cooking, food particles can block the steam release vent. Instant Pot has a structured vent shield that prevents blocking the steam release.

5) Automatic Temperature Control

Based on the type of food being cooked, the thermostat under the inner pot regulates the temperature and keep it within a safe range.

6) High-Temperature Warning

Sometimes over heating can be a possibility in case inner pot is missing, no proper contact with the heating element, or inner pot facing the heat dissipation problem. Under this scenario, Instant Pot will stop heating when the temperature is over a certain limit.

7) Power Protection & Extreme Temperature

Instant Pot disconnects the power itself if the temperature is very high, i.e. 169°C-172°C or 336°F-341.6°F, and if the electrical current is extremely high. To Instant Pot, an extremely high electrical current is an unsafe situation.

8) Automatic Pressure Control

The pressure sensor mechanism in Instant Pot keeps the operating pressure between 10.12psi-11.6 psi or 70kPa-80kPa.

9) Pressure Regulator Protection

If the pressure inside Instant Pot exceeds 105kPa (15.23 psi), the steam release will be pushed up to allow the steam being released to bring down the pressure inside the pot.

10) Excess Pressure Protection

Instant Pot activates its internal protection mechanism if the pressure regulator protection is malfunctioned or the pressure becomes too high. In this situation, it will create a gap between the lid and the inner pot by shifting the inner pot downwards. This will make the steam to be released from the gap into the internal chamber and heating will be stopped.

The more you cook using Instant pot, the more you will understand how it works and precautions that you should take while using Instant Pot.

Here is the list of 10 most common mistakes that a new Instant Pot user make so that you can avoid the unnecessary frustrations and stress while you use your new Instant Pot.

1. Pouring in Ingredients without Placing the Inner Pot Back into Instant Pot

Mistake: We all know Kitchen can be chaotic sometime and it's not surprising that, accidently, we can pour all ingredients into Instant Pot without the Inner Pot. This happens more frequently and almost to all of us.

Solution: Every time you remove the Inner Pot, place a glass lid, wooden spoon, silicone mat on top of Instant Pot. This can help preventing unnecessary damage to your Instant Pot!

2. Overfilling Instant Pot

Mistake: There are many instances where a new user filled Instant Pot with liquid and food up to the Max line that has led to the clogging of the Venting Knob.

Solution: Be careful of the fact that the Max Line printed on the Inner Pot is not for Pressure Cooking.

Pressure Cooking: 2/3 full max

Pressure Cooking Ingredients that Expands During Cooking (such as beans, dried vegetables, and grains): 1/2 full max

If the pot is overfilled by accident, just don't panic. Make sure you are using Natural Pressure Release to stay clean and safe.

3. Use Quick Release When It is Overfilled or in Case of Foamy Food

Mistake: New users are generally unsure when to use Natural Pressure Release and Quick Pressure Release. Instant Pot splatters if a user uses Quick Release while cooking foamy food, such as, beans or grains.

Solution #1: Use Natural Release when the pot is overfilled or for foamy food.

Solution #2: If you are cooking, for example, pasta that required Quick Release, then you have to release the pressure gradually.

Remember, not to turn the Venting Knob all the way to Venting Position in order to release pressure. You will find the initial release to be the strongest, so release the pressure gradually by turning the venting knob just a little with a wooden spoon or your hand until you hear a hissing sound.

4. Set Cooking Time by Pressing the Timer Button

Mistake: The Timer button on Instant Pot can be mistaken for setting the cooking time. Please note that the Timer button is for delayed cooking only.

Solution: Before you presume that your Instant Pot is not working properly, check to see whether the Timer button is on, showing the green color. If that is the case, press the Keep Warm/Cancel button to restart.

5. Forget to Turn the Venting Knob to Sealing Position

Mistake: It's very common to forget to turn the Venting Knob to the Sealing Position when cooking, especially if you are trying to use Instant Pot in the beginning.

Solution: Every time you start cooking in Instant Pot, make sure to turn the Venting Knob to Sealing Position. Make sure that the Floating Valve is popped up.

6. Put Instant Pot on the Stovetop and Accidentally Turned the Dial

Mistake: Due to limited counter space or convenience, many users put their Instant Pot on the stovetop. Sometimes, this can lead to melted burnt Instant Pot bottom due to many reasons.

Solution: Make sure that you don't put Instant Pot directly on the stovetop. You can use a wooden board between Instant Pot and stovetop to prevent this disaster.

7. Cooking Liquid: Not Enough Liquid/Too Thick

Mistake: A new user might find it tough to figure out how much cooking liquid to use. Instant Pot will not generate enough steam to build the pressure if there is not enough cooking liquid or the liquid is too thick.

Solutions: It is recommended to a new user to use 1 cup of total liquid till they are comfortable with the machine or unless stated otherwise in a recipe.

Always add a thickener such as flour, cornstarch, potato starch, or arrowhead after the pressure cooking cycle.

8. Forget to Put the Sealing Ring Back in the Lid before Cooking

Mistake: Many users forget to place the silicone sealing ring back into Instant Pot lid after washing it.

Solution: Before you close the lid, make sure that the sealing ring is properly installed every time.

9. Use Rice Button for Cooking All Types of Rice

Mistake: Many new users sometimes don't see satisfactory results while cooking rice in Instant Pot using the Rice button.

Solution: Each type of rice has its specific rice ratio and cooking time. For better results, you can use the Manual button to have more control on cooking method and time.

10. Use Hot Liquid in a Recipe that Calls for Cold Liquid

Mistake: Some new users pour hot liquid in Instant Pot for cooking and it results in meals being undercooked. This is because the hot water shortens the cooking time and Instant Pot will take the shorter time to build pressure and thus the food may come out as undercooked.

Solution: Always use cold liquid for cooking or adjust the cooking time as per the recipe.

LOW CARB INSTANT POT COOKBOOK
INSTANT POT SHREDDED TACO BEEF
INGREDIENTS

- 2 lb. flank steak

- 1 tbsp. olive oil

- 1 white or yellow onion, sliced

- 2 cloves garlic, smashed

- salt and pepper, to taste

- 1 tsp. ground cumin

- 1/2 tsp. chili powder

- 1/4 cup salsa verde

- 1/4 cup chicken broth

- 1 tbsp. tomato paste

- 1/8 tsp. cayenne pepper (optional for spicy!)

INSTRUCTIONS

- Turn instant pot on "saute" mode.

- Add oil in the bottom of the pot and when warm, add onions and saute with a little salt and pepper until tender, about 5 minutes.

- Add in the garlic and cut flank steak into smaller hunks of meat (about 6 inch hunks) and season them well with salt and pepper all over.

- While still on the "saute" function. Add the steak and sear on each side until browned, about 2-3 minutes per side.

- Add in the salsa verde, broth, chili powder, cumin, and tomato paste. Toss using tongs to combine evenly.

- Press the "Cancel/keep warm" button.

• Now press the "Manual" button and turn it down to 45 minutes on high pressure.

• Seal and cook until time is done. When time is complete, turn the valve from sealing to venting to release the pressure quickly.

• When pressure is released, using tongs transfer the meat onto a cutting board and using two forks, shred the meat. Discard all but about 1/4 cup of the excess liquid in the instant pot. Place the meat back into the instant pot and toss in the liquid until it is all soaked up.

• Serve taco salad style, in tacos, on nachos, stuffed in peppers, or however you please!! Enjoy!

PALEO BEEF BRISKET PHO (AN INSTANT POT RECIPE)

INGREDIENTS

- 1.75 - 2 lbs Beef brisket

- 1-1.25 lbs beef shank soup bones, , beef knuckle bones, or a combination

- 1 ¼ cups dry shiitake mushrooms*, (rehydrate overnight in room temperature water)

- 3 loose carrots, roughly chopped*

- 1 medium size yellow onion, peeled but not sliced (leave it as a whole)

- 1 large size leek, roughly diced into segments

- Water

- 2 ½ tsp fine sea salt*

- 1 tbsp Red Boat fish sauce

- 1 tsp five spice powder, (optional)

- Tea bags or cheese cloth

Pho Aroma Combo:

- 2 fat thumb size ginger, (scrub clean, no need to peel)

- 4 star anise

- 2 cinnamon sticks

- 8 green cardamom

- 3 medium size shallots

- 4-5 cilantro roots, (alt. 1 ½ tsp coriander seeds)

Garnish:

- Lime wedges

- Baby bok choy

- Bean sprouts

- Red or green fresno chili peppers

- Mint leaves

- Asian/Thai basil, (optional)

- Cilantro, (optional)

- Hot chili pepper sauce, (optional)

INSTRUCTIONS

Pre-Cooking:

- Soak the dry shiitake mushrooms overnight in room temperature water. If rush on time, soak in warm temperature water until the mushrooms are soft and tender.

- Pre-boil the bones and brisket: add the bones and brisket to a large stockpot and cover with water. Bring the water to boil over high heat, then reduce to medium and simmer for 10 more minutes. Rinse the bones and meat over room temperature tap water.* Set aside. Discard the broth.

- Grill the ingredients under "Pho Aroma Combo" in a cast iron over medium heat. No oil added. Rotate and flip the ingredients frequently until you can smell a nice and lovely fragrant. Be careful not to burn the aroma combo. Slightly charred outer surface is okay but not burnt.

- Slice the mushrooms. Save the mushroom water. Roughly dice leek. Add aroma combo and leeks to large tea bags or cheesecloth tied with a string.*

Instant Pot Cooking:

- In a 6-quart size instant pot, add beef bones, brisket (fatty side up)*, slicedd shiitake, diced carrots, aroma combo, onion, and leeks (in tea bags). Strain the mushroom water as you add the liquid to the pot. Fill the pot with more tap water until it reaches the 4 liter mark. Close the lid in Sealing position - Press Soup - Adjust to 40 minutes/High pressure/More.

- Allow the instant pot come to natural pressure release (valve dropped), discard the whole onion and aroma combo in tea bags.

• Remove the brisket and soak it in cold water for at least 10 minutes. This will prevent the meat from turning dark color. Discard aroma & leek tea bags, yellow onion, and beef bones. Season the broth with 2 ½ tsp fine sea salt, 1 tbsp fish sauce, and 1 tsp five spice powder (optional).

• Thin slice the brisket in 45 degree angle and against the grain. Ladle the broth over bean sprouts, carrots, mushrooms, mint leaves, Asian basil, chili peppers, and sliced brisket. Serve hot with lime wedges.

Low carb Instant Pot Greek Cauliflower Rice

INGREDIENTS

- 1 small head cauliflower, trimmed and cut into quarters
- 2 tablespoons olive oil, divided
- ½ cup diced red onion
- 1 tablespoon minced garlic
- 1 cup halved grape tomatoes
- ½ cup chopped English cucumber
- ½ cup halved kalamata olives
- ½ cup crumbled feta cheese
- ¼ cup chopped fresh parsley
- Grated zest and juice of 1 lemon
- ¼ teaspoon fine sea salt
- ¼ teaspoon black pepper
- ¼ cup chopped walnuts, toasted if desired

Direction

1. Pour 1 cup water into the Instant Pot. Place the cauliflower on a trivet with handles and lower the trivet into the pot. Secure the lid on the pot and close the pressure-release valve. Set the pot to High Pressure for 0 minutes (see note). At the end of the cooking time, quick-release the pressure. Transfer the cauliflower to a large bowl and set aside. Discard the liquid from the pot and wipe dry.

2. Select Sauté on the Instant Pot. When the pot is hot, add 1 tablespoon of the olive oil. Add the onion and garlic to the hot oil and cook until tender, about 4 minutes. Select Cancel. Return the cauliflower to the pot and use a potato masher or wooden spoon to break the chunks into small, rice-size pieces.

3. Transfer the cauliflower to a serving bowl. Add the tomatoes, cucumber, olives, feta, parsley, lemon zest and lemon juice, and toss gently to combine. Season with the salt and pepper. Just before serving, fold in the walnuts and drizzle with the remaining 1 tablespoon olive oil.

NOTE: Use the "0 minutes" cooking time for foods that don't need a lot of time to cook, like cauliflower florets. The pressure cooker will still build pressure, and as it does, it will cook the food (which will also continue to cook while the pressure is being released).

Instant Pot low carb Indian Butter Chicken

INGREDIENTS

- 2 pounds boneless, skinless chicken thighs
- 1 teaspoon plus ¾ teaspoon fine Himalayan pink salt, divided
- ½ teaspoon freshly ground black pepper
- 4 tablespoons butter or ghee, divided
- 2 garlic cloves, minced
- 1 small onion, chopped
- 1 jalapeño pepper, finely chopped (seeded if desired)
- 1 tablespoon garam masala
- 2 teaspoons minced fresh ginger
- 1 teaspoon ground cumin
- 1 teaspoon ground turmeric
- 1 cup heavy cream or coconut cream
- ¼ cup chopped fresh cilantro

Direction

1. Season the chicken with 1 teaspoon of the salt and the pepper. Select Sauté on the Instant Pot. Add 1 tablespoon of the butter and the minced garlic. When the butter is melted, add half the chicken in a single layer. Cook until browned on both sides, 6 to 8 minutes, turning once. Remove the chicken from the pot and repeat with the remaining chicken and 1 additional tablespoon of butter.

2. Add the onion and jalapeño to the pot. Cook, stirring often, until tender, about 3 minutes. Stir in the garam masala, ginger, cumin, turmeric and ¾ teaspoon pink salt. Cook for about 1 minute. Return the chicken to the pot. Select Cancel.

3. Secure the lid on the pot and close the pressure-release valve. Set the pot to High Pressure for 10 minutes. At the end of the cooking time, allow a

natural pressure release for 10 minutes, then quick-release the remaining pressure.

4. Stir in the cream, cilantro and the remaining butter.

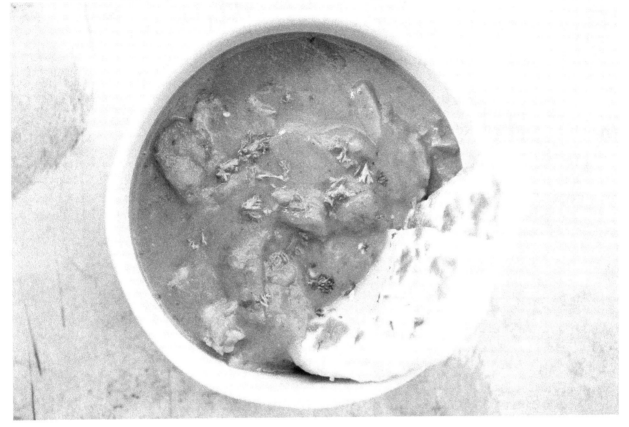

Low carb Instant Pot Sausage-Kale Soup

INGREDIENTS

- 2 tablespoons extra-virgin olive oil

- ½ pound uncured sausage, sliced into ½-inch-thick rounds

- ½ cup diced yellow onion

- 2 tablespoons minced garlic

- ½ teaspoon smoked paprika

- ¼ to ½ teaspoon crushed red-pepper flakes, to taste

- 4 cups chicken broth

- 2 cups cauliflower rice

- 3 cups chopped fresh kale

- ¼ teaspoon fine sea salt

- ¼ teaspoon freshly ground black pepper

Direction

1. Select Sauté on the Instant Pot. When the pot is hot, add the olive oil. Add the sausage, onion, garlic, paprika and pepper flakes to the hot oil and cook, stirring often, until the onion softens and the sausage starts to brown, about 5 minutes. Select Cancel. Add the broth and cauliflower rice.

2. Secure the lid on the pot and close the pressure-release valve. Set the pot to High Pressure for 5 minutes. At the end of the cooking time, quick-release the pressure.

3. Stir in the kale, salt and pepper. Let the soup stand for 5 minutes to soften the kale before serving.

INSTANT POT CHICKEN AND "RICE" SOUP

INGREDIENTS

- 2 tbsp olive oil

- 1 cup diced yellow onion (or 1/2 large onion)

- 3/4 cup loosely chopped celery (or 2 stalks)

- 1 cup loosely chopped carrot (or 1 large carrot)

- 2 cloves garlic, minced

- 1 tsp kosher salt

- 1/2 tsp black pepper

- 4 cups low sodium chicken broth

- 1 lb chicken breast, boneless skinless

- 1 tsp fresh thyme or 1/2 tsp dried thyme

- 1 bay leaf

- 4 cups baby spinach

- 1/3 cup fresh riced cauliflower, not frozen

- Juice of 1/2 lemon

INSTRUCTIONS

- Turn Instant Pot to the "sautee" function and heat 2 tbsp of olive oil. Once hot, add the onions, celery, carrots, garlic, salt and pepper. Sautee, stirring occasionally, for 5 minutes or until vegetables are slightly tender.

- Then, press the "cancel" button on the Instant Pot. Add the chicken broth, chicken breast, thyme and bay leaf. Secure lid and seal vent. Press the "manual" button and select the high pressure setting. Set time to 15 minutes.

- When the cooking time is up, turn the vent to the venting mode and release the pressure manually. Once pressure if fully released, carefully remove lid. Using tongs, transfer chicken breast to cutting board. Shred chicken using two forks and then place shredded chicken in soup. Stir in baby spinach, until just wilted. Taste soup and adjust seasonings, if desired.

• Spoon riced cauliflower into the bottom of a small bowl. Ladle soup over riced cauliflower (don't worry it will cook in a few moments with the hot broth). Finish with lemon juice.

• Serve and enjoy!

INSTANT POT GARLIC PARMESAN SPAGHETTI SQUASH

Ingredients

- 1 large spaghetti squash
- 3 tablespoons olive oil
- 8 cloves Garlic, sliced thinly
- 1 teaspoon red pepper flakes
- ½ cup slivered almonds, or other nuts of choice
- 4 cups fresh spinach, chopped
- 1 teaspoon Kosher Salt
- 1 cup shredded parmesan cheese
- 1.5 cups water, for the Instant Pot

Instructions

- Using the tip of a sharp, short knife, pierce the spaghetti squash in 7-8 places.

- Put 1.5 cups of water into the Instant Pot. Place a steamer rack into the pot. Place the pierced spaghetti squash on the rack.

- Close the lid and set the Instant Pot to cook on HIGH PRESSURE for 7 minutes. At the end of the cooking time, allow the pot to rest undisturbed for 10 minutes.

- Remove the squash and cut it open lengthwise, so that you can have long spaghetti-like strands. Put away half for another use.

- Drag a fork along the squash to get long strands of spaghetti squash. Measure out 4 cups and set the rest aside for another use (like eating all the time at any excuse.) Save the squash shell since you will be serving your elegant creation in it.

- Empty out the Instant Pot and wipe dry.

- Press Sauté. When the pot is hot, add oil. To the hot oil, add garlic, red pepper, and slivered almonds or pine nuts. Toast for 1 minute without letting the garlic burn. Add in the spinach and salt and stir.

• Add in spaghetti squash.

• Sprinkle with parmesan cheese just before serving.

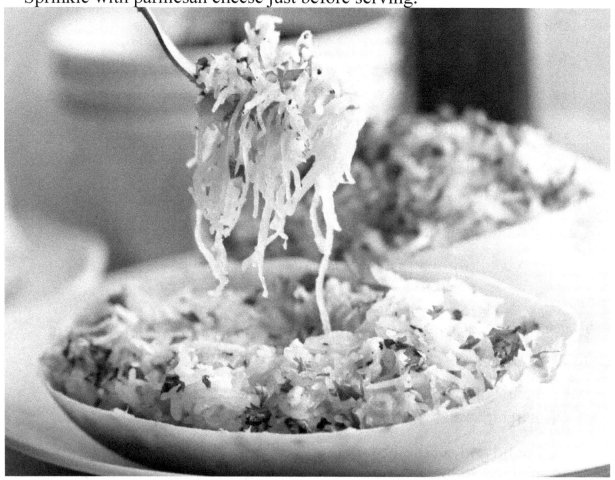

LOW CARB BUFFALO CHICKEN SOUP RECIPE – INSTANT POT PRESSURE COOKER

INGREDIENTS

- 1 tbsp Olive oil

- 1/2 large Onion (diced)

- 1/2 cup Celery (diced)

- 4 cloves Garlic (minced)

- 1 lb Shredded chicken (cooked)

- 4 cup Chicken bone broth (or any chicken broth)

- 3 tbsp Buffalo sauce (or 2 tbsp for less heat)

- 6 oz Cream cheese (at room temperature, cubed)

- 1/2 cup Half & half (or heavy cream)

Instructions

• Press the Saute button on the Instant Pot. Add the oil, chopped onion, and celery. Cook for about 5-10 minutes, stirring occasionally, until onions are translucent and start to brown.

• Add garlic. Saute for about a minute, until fragrant. Press the Off button.

• Add the shredded chicken, broth, and buffalo sauce.

• Cover and seal the Instant Pot. Press the Soup button and adjust time to 5 minutes. After cooking is complete, let pressure release naturally for 5 minutes, then switch to quick release and open the lid.

• Ladle about a cup of liquid (without chicken) from the edge of the Instant Pot and pour into a blender. Add the cubed cream cheese. Puree until smooth. (If it's hard to blend, you can add a little more liquid.)

• Pour the mixture back into the Instant Pot. Add the half & half or heavy cream. Stir until smooth.

Instant Pot Low carb Corned Beef Brisket

INGREDIENTS

- 2-3 pound Corned Beef Brisket

- 1.5 cups Water, filtered

- Garlic

- Onion

- organic bay leaves

INSTRUCTIONS

- Place the spice pack that comes with your corned beef brisket, bay leaf, onion and garlic with water in the bottom of your pressure cooker.

- Place brisket on a rack above the liquid. If you don't have rack that's ok, you'll just want to pick the spices off the brisket when done.

- Cook under high or standard pressure for 1 hour and 30 minutes.

- Can be quick depressurized or naturally depressurized.

- Remove brisket from the cooker, slice against the grain. Enjoy!

No Bean Whole30 Keto Chili In The Instant Pot

INGREDIENTS

- 1½ Tbsp Olive oil, divided

- ½ Cup Onion, diced

- 1 Red pepper, diced

- ½ Cup Celery sliced

- 1 Tbsp Garlic, minced

- 1 Lb Grass-fed 85% lean Ground beef

- 4 tsp Chile powder

- 1 Tbsp Smoked paprika

- ¼ tsp Cayenne pepper

- 1/8 tsp Ground Allspice

- 1 Can Fire roasted diced tomatoes (14oz)

- 1 Can Crushed tomatoes (14 oz)

- ½ Cup Water

- 2 Tbsp Tomato paste

- 1 tsp Sea salt

- Pinch of pepper

- 2 Bay leaves

- ¼ Cup Parsley minced

INSTRUCTIONS

- Pour 1 Tbsp of the oil in your Instant Pot and turn it to saute mode. Once hot, saute the onion, pepper, celery and garlic until they begin to soften, about 3 minutes.

- Add the remaining oil, along with the beef and cook until it begins to turn brown, about 3-4 minutes. Drain the excess fat.

• Add in the chili powder, paprika, cayenne and Allspice and cook until the beef is totally brown and no longer pink, about 3-4 minutes.

• Add all the remaining ingredients, except the parsley, and stir until well combined. Cover the Instant Pot (make sure it's set to sealing) and turn it to manual mode (it should immediately be set for high pressure) set it for 10 minutes. Once cooked, let it steam release naturally.

• Once the steam is released, remove the lid and turn it to saute mode. Cook for 2-4 minutes, stirring frequently, until some of the water is evaporated.

• Stir in the parsley and DEVOUR!

Low carb Bacon Cheeseburger Soup – Instant Pot Recipe

Ingredients

- 1 pound 85% lean ground beef

- ½ medium onion, sliced

- ½ (14.5-ounce) can fire-roasted tomatoes

- 3 cups Beef Broth

- ¼ cup cooked crumbled bacon

- 1 tablespoon chopped pickle jalapenos

- 1 teaspoon salt

- ½ teaspoon pepper

- ½ teaspoon garlic powder

- 2 teaspoons Worcestershire sauce

- 4 ounces cream cheese

- 1 cup sharp cheddar cheese, shredded

- 1 pickle spear, diced

Instructions

• Press the Saute button and add ground beef. Brown beef halfway and add onion. Continue cooking beef until no pink remains. Press the Cancel button. Add tomatoes, broth, bacon, jalapenos, salt, pepper, garlic powder, and Worcestershire sauce, and stir. Place cream cheese on top in middle.

• Click lid closed. Press the Soup button and adjust time for 15 minutes. When timer beeps, quick-release the pressure. Top with diced pickles and garnish with shredded cheddar.

Instant Pot Chicken Tikka Masala

INGREDIENTS

Chicken

- 3 large boneless skinless chicken breasts about 2 pounds, diced
- 1 cup plain yogurt non-dairy if paleo, on Whole30, or need dairy-free. Can omit entirely
- 1 tsp. turmeric
- 2 tsp. garam masala
- 1 Tbsp. lemon juice about half a lemon
- 2 tsp. black pepper
- ¼ tsp. dried ginger

Sauce

- ¼ cup ghee or butter 4 Tbsp., use ghee if paleo or on Whole30
- 1 medium white onion diced
- 2 serrano chiles minced (deseeded for mild, seeds left in for medium/hot)
- 5 garlic cloves minced
- 1½ Tbsp. fresh ginger grated
- 4½ tsp. garam masala
- 1 tsp. paprika
- 1 15- ounce can tomato sauce
- 1 green bell pepper deseeded and sliced into strips
- 1 Tbsp. dried fenugreek leaves
- salt to taste
- 1-2 cups coconut cream just the solid white part from a can of coconut milk or cream

Equipment Needed

• Instant Pot

To Serve

steamed cauliflower rice or basmati rice use cauliflower rice for paleo or Whole30

fresh cilantro chopped

INSTRUCTIONS

• In a medium bowl, whisk together all marinade ingredients besides chicken. Toss chicken in marinade to coat well. Cover and refrigerate at least 1 hour, up to overnight.

• In the Instant Pot in Sauté Mode, Normal Heat, heat the ghee or butter. Add onion and cook until softened, about 4-5 minutes. Reduce heat to Low Heat. Add serrano chiles, garlic, and ginger, and cook, stirring occasionally, until a nice, even toffee-brown color, about 10 minutes. Add 1-2 teaspoons water as needed if you notice the mixture sticking or drying out. If you cook this part over Normal Heat, monitor the mixture very closely. It will burn if you don't watch it well!

• When mixture is a toffee brown color, add garam masala and paprika; stir well. Cook a few minutes, or until fragrant, adding a couple tablespoons of water to reduce sticking, if necessary.

• Add the tomato sauce and stir well; transfer mixture to the blender and blend until smooth. Return sauce to pot and simmer for 15-25 minutes over Normal Heat or until thick like a paste, rather than like a sauce.

• Add chicken, sliced bell pepper, fenugreek leaves, and salt. Secure lid and cook on Manual High Pressure for 6 minutes. Carefully Quick Release.

• Add the coconut cream and stir until smooth. Taste and correct seasonings, adding more salt or fenugreek leaves as necessary. Serve over steamed cauliflower or basmati rice and top with plenty of chopped fresh cilantro.

Healthy Chicken Pot Pie Soup

INGREDIENTS

- 2 large boneless skinless chicken breasts cut into bite-sized chunks
- 2 Tbsp. ghee or olive oil
- 1 onion diced, 1 cup
- 3 carrots diced, 1 cup
- 3 stalks celery sliced, 1 cup
- 5-6 cloves garlic minced
- 1 pound red potatoes diced
- 2 cups chicken broth or stock
- 1 cup full-fat canned coconut cream or milk
- 1 cup cashews
- 2 Tbsp. fresh thyme leaves
- 1½ tsp. salt
- 1½ tsp. dried sage
- freshly cracked black pepper
- fresh parsley leaves chopped, for garnish

INSTRUCTIONS

- Turn Instant Pot on Sauté mode. Melt ghee in the pot, then add onion, carrots, and celery, stirring regularly. Cook until onions are soft, then add garlic and cook, stirring constantly, until fragrant, about 30 seconds to 1 minute.

- Add potatoes, chicken broth, chicken, dried sage, and fresh thyme to Instant Pot. Secure lid with the valve in Sealing position and cook Manual High Pressure for 10 minutes.

- Meanwhile, add coconut milk and cashews to a high-speed blender. Blend until very, very smooth.

• When time is up, Quick Release, then stir in the coconut-cashew mixture and add salt and freshly cracked black pepper to taste.

BALSAMIC CHICKEN [INSTANT POT]

INGREDIENTS

olive oil cooking spray

- 1–2lbs boneless, skinless chicken breast

- 1 28oz can of diced or crushed tomatoes (I love it with either!)

- ½ red onion, thinly sliced

- 2 cloves of garlic, minced

- ½ cup balsamic vinegar

- ½ tsp dried basil

- ½ tsp dried oregano

- ½ tsp garlic powder

- salt

- pepper

- zoodles (optional)

INSTRUCTIONS

- Spray Instant Pot with cooking spray and use Saute button to saute onions until they become soft and translucent. Add minced garlic and saute for an additional minute.

- Add chicken, tomatoes, balsamic vinegar, and spices to pot.

- Set to manual/pressure cook for 15 minutes. After cook time, do a full natural release (about 10 minutes).

- Shred chicken and serve with sauce and zoodles* or pasta!

*I don't even cook the zoodles – I allow it to steam in the sauce, but feel free to saute also!

Note: The cook time for the chicken used to be 10 minutes with QR. Now, I find that 15 minutes with a full natural release works better!

INSTANT POT SHRIMP WITH TOMATOES AND FETA | GREEK SHRIMP SAGANAKI

Ingredients

Cook Together

- 2 tablespoons (2 tablespoons) Butter

- 1 tablespoon (1 tablespoon) Garlic

- ½ teaspoon (0.5 teaspoon) Red Pepper Flakes, adjust to taste

- 1.5 cups (32 g) onions, chopped

- 1 14.5-oz (1 14.5-oz) Canned Tomatoes

- 1 teaspoon (1 teaspoon) Dried Oregano

- 1 teaspoons (1 teaspoons) Kosher Salt

- 1 pound (453.59 g) Frozen Raw Shrimp, 21-25 count, shelled

Add after cooking

- 1 cup (150 g) crumbled feta cheese

- ½ cup (67.5 g) sliced black olives

- ¼ cup (15 g) Chopped Parsley

Instructions

For the Instant Pot

- Turn your Instant Pot or Pressure cooker to Sauté and once it is hot, add the butter. Let it melt a little and then add garlic and red pepper flakes.

- Add in onions, tomatoes, oregano and salt.

- Pour in the frozen shrimp.

- Set your Instant pot to LOW pressure 1 minute.

- Once the pot is done cooking, release all pressure immediately.

- Mix in the shrimp with the rest of the lovely tomato broth.

• Allow it to cool slightly. Right before serving, sprinkle the feta cheese, olives, and parsley.

• This dish makes a soupy broth, so it's great for dipping buttered french bread into, or eat over rice, or riced cauliflower.

INSTANT POT ORANGE CHICKEN RECIPE

Ingredients

- ½ cup chicken broth

- ¼ cup freshly squeezed orange juice

- ½ cup seasoned rice vinegar

- ½ cup soy sauce or gluten free alternative

- 2 tablespoons honey

- 2 cloves garlic minced or pressed

- 1 tablespoon grated orange zest about 1 orange worth

- 1 teaspoon red pepper flakes more or less to taste

- ¼ teaspoon ground ginger

- ¼ teaspoon black pepper

- 1½ pounds uncooked boneless skinless chicken breasts I use 3 (8 oz) chicken breasts

- 2 tablespoons cornstarch

- 2-4 tablespoons freshly squeezed orange juice

- Green onion sliced for garnish

- Cilantro chopped for garnish

- Sesame seeds for garnish

- Cauliflower rice, brown rice, etc for serving

Instructions

- Grease Instant Pot with cooking spray. Set aside.

- Whisk together broth, 1/4 cup orange juice, vinegar, soy sauce, honey, garlic, orange zest, red pepper flakes, ground ginger, and black pepper.

- Pour half into Instant Pot.

- Place in chicken breasts.

- Pour remaining sauce over chicken breasts.

- Cover and lock lid (ensure steam releasing handle is pointing to "sealing").

- Cook using the manual button (set to high pressure) and adjust timer on the Instant Pot to 12 minutes.*

- The Instant Pot will beep when it's finished. Flip the valve to "venting" for a quick release.

- Remove chicken and set aside.

- In a small bowl, whisk together cornstarch with 2-4 tablespoons of orange juice.***

- Whisk that mixture into the Instant Pot.

- Press the saute button on the Instant Pot and bring the sauce to a simmer.

- Add chicken back in and simmer until the sauce has thickened, about 5 minutes.

- Shred the chicken directly in the pot as the sauce is thickening.

- Taste and re-season, if necessary and serve

PUMPKIN CHICKEN CURRY (INSTANT POT)

- 3 tbsp olive oil

- 3 garlic cloves

- ½ onion

- 2 lbs chicken breast

- ¼ can pumpkin puree usually 1 can is 15oz

- 1 cup chicken stock/broth

- ½ cup coconut milk

- 1 tbsp tomato paste

- ½ tsp cumin

- 1 tbsp curry powder

- ½ tsp smoked paprika

- ½ tsp cayenne pepper

- ½ tsp salt or to taste

Instructions

MAKE IT IN THE INSTANT POT

- First, chop your onions and mince the garlic.

- Cut the chicken breast into medium-sized cubes.

- Turn on your instant pot to sauté mode and warm up the olive oil.

- Add in the onions and garlic and stir them until they are golden brown.

- Next, add in the chicken breast, tomato paste, and spices and mix them well.

- Add the chicken stock and pumpkin puree and stir it again.

- Set your instant pot to manual mode and adjust it to high pressure for 5 minutes.

- Once it's done, let the pressure naturally release all the way.

• Remove the lid and add coconut milk at the end and allow the pumpkin chicken curry to thicken as it simmers.

• Taste for salt and adjust according to your preference.

• Top it off with some parsley or any herb of your choice and serve!

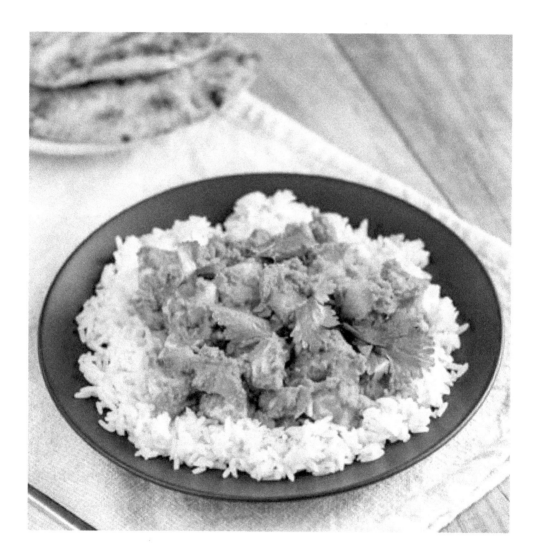

INGREDIENTS

- 1 lb lamb stew meat, cut into 1 inch cubes (shoulder or leg meat works great)

- 1 teaspoon kosher salt

- ½ teaspoon black pepper

- 2 tbsp arrowroot flour (you can sub tapioca or regular flour here, too)

- 2 tbsp extra virgin olive oil

- 1 cup carrots, sliced diagonally about ½ inch thick (or 2 large carrots)

- ½ cup celery, diced large (or 1 stalk)

- ¾ cup yellow onion, diced (or ½ medium onion)

- 2 cloves garlic, minced

- ¼ tsp chili flakes (optional)

- 1 tbsp tomato paste

- 1 cup red wine

- 1 tsp fresh thyme leaves (4-5 sprigs)

- 2 cups russet potato, peeled and chopped into 1-inch cubes

- 1 bay leaf

- 1 cup beef broth + ¼ cup

- ½ tsp freshly chopped rosemary leaves (about 1 sprig)

INSTRUCTIONS

- Pat dry the cubed lamb meat and place in a large bowl with the salt, pepper, and 1 tablespoon arrowroot flour. Toss until evenly coated.

- Turn the Instant Pot on the sauté function with olive oil. When hot, in batches, sear the lamb meat until golden brown on all sides. About 2-3 minutes per side. Set browned meat aside and continue cooking until all meat is finished cooking.

• Add garlic, celery, carrot, onion and chili flakes (optional) to the Instant Pot (still on sauté function). Stir and sauté the veggies until softened, scraping any of the brown edges from the pot. About 3 minutes.

• Once vegetables are softened, add tomato past. Stir until veggies are coated. Add red wine and stir, scraping brown bits from bottom.

• Add the potato, lamb (plus any of its juices), thyme, rosemary, bay leaf and beef broth into the pot.

• Securely fasten the lid on top of the Instant Pot. Hit the cancel button then hit the meat/stew function. Lower the time to 40 minutes.

• When the cook time has complete, hit the 'cancel' button and release the pressure in the Instant pot manually by carefully turning the valve to "venting". Let vent until all the steam has released and carefully remove the lid.

• Turn the instant pot back onto the 'sauté' function. Meanwhile, in a small bowl combine the remaining 1 tablespoon of the arrowroot with the remaining 1/4 cup of beef broth. Whisk until the arrowroot has dissolved in the liquid, making a "slurry" that will help thicken the soup.

• With the sauté function on and while stirring, slowly pour the slurry into the soup, stirring, until the soup has thickened, about 2 minutes.

BBQ Instant Pot Whole Chicken

Ingredients

• [BBQ Rub]

• 4 Pound Whole Chicken

• 'Olive oil

• 1/3 Cup Apple Juice

• [Instant pot]

Instructions

• Prepare the bbq rub and massage it both under and over the skin.

• Drizzle some oil in your Instant Pot.

• Turn it on to the saute function and allow it to heat up.

• Place the whole chicken, breast side down, in the Instant Pot. If it is too big to lay down flat you'll have to brown the skin on the stove top in a large skillet.

• Cook for a few minutes until golden and turn over, browning the other side.

• You can leave the chicken in the pot, or we like to use the Trivet so it isn't sitting in the liquid.

• Pour in the liquids and close the lid.

• Set the Instant Pot to manual high pressure and cook for 30 minutes.

• Allow the Instant Pot to do a slow release for 5-10 minutes and then remove the lid and enjoy!

Instant Pot Cuban-style beef lettuce wraps

Ingredients

- 2 lb flank steak (cut into 2 inch pieces)
- 1 onion (sliced)
- 3 garlic cloves (sliced)
- 1 tbspn chopped fresh oregano (or 1 teaspoon dry)
- 1 can stewed tomatoes
- 2 red bell peppers sliced
- ½ cup beef broth
- ½ green olives sliced
- olive oil for the pot bottom
- salt and pepper to taste
- 1 butter lettuce head

Instructions

- Turn your instant pot on, switch on the saute mode. Add oil in the pot and when its smoking, add beef. Brown on each side, then add onions and garlic. Cook for 5 minutes.

- Add oregano, broth, scrape all brown bits from the bottom, using a wooden spoon. Stir in tomatoes, olives, salt and pepper.

- Close the lid and push on a stew button. Adjust to 25 minutes on high pressure.

- Quick release the pressure. Transfer beef on a cutting board and shred. Meanwhile turn on saute function on your instant pot, add sliced bell peppers and cook for about 15 minutes. until tender. Stir in beef.

- Wash and dry butter lettuce. Separate into single leaves. Add Shredded beef mixture in to every lettuce cup and serve.

Instant Pot Whole Roasted Cauliflower With Chimichurri Sauce

INGREDIENTS

- 1 medium sized head of cauliflower

For the Chimichurri

- 1 cup packed fresh italian parsley
- ½ cup packed cilantro
- ⅓ cup olive oil
- ⅓ cup red wine vinegar
- 2 garlic cloves
- ½ teaspoon crushed red pepper
- ½ teaspoon ground cumin
- ½ teaspoon salt

For serving: hummus, toasted pine nuts

INSTRUCTIONS

- Rinse and dry cauliflower. Cut off the bottom stalk, being careful not to remove so much of the core that the cauliflower can't hold it's shape. Tear off remaining green leaves.

- Add 1 cup of water to the pressure cooker pot and place trivet inside. Place cauliflower core side down on top of the trivet.

- Secure the lid and turn pressure release knob to a sealed position. Cook at high pressure for 1 minute (or 2 minutes if you like it very soft).

- While the cauliflower cooks, make chimichurri by putting all of the ingredients into a food processor or blender. Pulse until it's right in the middle of being chunky and smooth.

- Preheat oven broiler.

- When pressure cooking is complete, use a quick release.

• Gently place cauliflower on a baking sheet. Separate the florets just a little bit to create some spaces for the chimichurri to soak in to.

• Brush cauliflower generously with the chimichurri sauce. You want some of the sauce to soak into the cracks so that it will flavor the inside too. Reserve the extra for serving.

• Place cauliflower under the oven broiler until it gets browned and crisp. Depending on your broiler this could be anywhere from 3 – 7 minutes. Watch closely so it doesn't burn.

• To serve, make a bed of hummus on a plate or in a shallow bowl. Cut cauliflower into wedges or 1 inch steaks and place on top of the hummus. Drizzle with extra chimichurri sauce and sprinkle with toasted pine nuts. Enjoy!

Instant Pot Turmeric Tahini Chicken Soup

INGREDIENTS

- 1 Cup Onion, diced (115g)

- 1 Cup Carrots, Thinly sliced (113g)

- 1 tsp Turmeric

- 1 tsp Fresh ginger, minced

- ½ tsp Ground coriander

- ¼ tsp Cinnamon

- ½ tsp Sea salt + more to taste

- 3 Cups Chicken stock (not sodium reduced)

- ½ Lb Boneless, skinless chicken breast

- ½ Cup Light coconut milk

- 2½ Tbsp Tahini

- 2 Cups Baby spinach, tightly packed

INSTRUCTIONS

- Place all the ingredients, up to the chicken, in the Instant Pot and stir to combine. Lay the chicken breast on top.

- Cover, set to sealing and cook on manual high pressure for 15 mins. Let steam release naturally when done.

- Remove the chicken from the pot and shred it with 2 forks. Place it back into the pot.

- Pour 1 cup of the soup (including any shredded chicken) into a high-powered blender and blend until smooth. Pour back into the soup.

- Add the coconut milk, tahini and spinach and stir. You can cover the pot and turn to sautee mode for a few minutes to let the spinach wilt, if it doesn't on it's own.

- Adjust the salt to taste and DEVOUR!

INSTANT POT STEAK FAJITAS RECIPE

Ingredients

- 1 lb Skirt steak (or flank steak; sliced thinly against the grain)

- 2 tbsp Fajita seasoning mix (divided)

- 1 tbsp Avocado oil

- 2 large Bell peppers (sliced into thin strips)

- 1 medium Onion (sliced into thin half moons)

- ½ cup Beef bone broth (or any broth of choice)

- 2 tbsp Lime juice

Instructions

- Toss the steak in a tablespoon of fajita seasoning.

- Press the "Saute" button on the Instant Pot and adjust temperature to "More" (by pressing "Saute" repeatedly until the screen says "More"). Add a tablespoon of oil and half the steak in a single layer. Saute for about 1-2 minutes per side, not to cook through but just to brown the steak. Remove and repeat with the remaining steak. Add the steak that was cooked from the first batch back to the pot.

- Add the vegetables and sprinkle with remaining fajita seasoning. Stir vegetables if needed to coat in seasoning. Add the broth and lime juice.

- Close the lid and close the vent to the Sealing position. Press the "Manual" button and set to 2 minutes on High pressure. Use the Quick Release to release pressure immediately.

No Noodle Lasagna

Ingredients

- 1 pound ground beef

- 2 cloves garlic minced

- 1 small onion

- 1½ cups ricotta cheese

- ½ cup Parmesan cheese

- 1 large egg use one more for a thicker lasagna

- 1 jar marinara sauce 25 ounces

- 8 ounces mozzarella sliced

Instructions

- On sauté setting, brown the ground beef with the garlic and onion.

- While the meat is browning, combine the ricotta cheese with the Parmesan and egg in a small mixing bowl.

- Drain grease and remove meat mixture from Instant Pot.

- In a medium size bowl mix meat mixture with 25 ounce jar of marinara (reserve ½ c for the top).

- Next, using a round dish that fits within your Instant Pot (A springform pan with aluminum foil to catch any drippings works) layer half of your lasagna meat, mozzarella and ricotta cheese mixture repeating for a second time until no ingredients remain. Top with ½ c of reserved marinara sauce.

- Place sling in Instant Pot over rack and pour in 1 cup of water.

- Set dish in instant pot. Cover loosely with aluminum foil if desired to keep condensation from dripping on the lasagna.

- Attach lid, close valve, and cook on high pressure for 9 minutes.

- Vent steam, remove the lid and serve.

THAI GREEN CURRY RECIPE

INGREDIENTS

- 1.5-2 lbs boneless/skinless chicken thighs, or breasts or a combination

- 2.5-3 tbsp Mae Ploy green curry paste, see notes

- 1 cup chicken stock

- 6 whole dried kaffir lime leaves , or 3 fresh kaffir lime leaves, optional, see notes for alternative

- 2 tbsp fish sauce

- 140 gram bamboo shoots, liquid drained

- 1 cup coconut milk cream, or use the top cream part of a canned 14 oz. full fat coconut milk

- 3-4 tbsp nut butter of choice, or sunbutter for nut-free

- Half one whole lime juice or to taste, plus extra for garnish

Optional roasted vegetable choices:

- 2 cups eggplants, diced

- 2 cups butternut squash, diced

- 1 cup carrots, diced

- 1 tsp coarse sea salt

- 3 tbsp olive oil

Serving:

- Sugar snap peas or snow peas, sliced lengthwise, as much as you like

- Cilantro, garnish, optional

INSTRUCTIONS

For Meal prep -

- In a gallon size freezer friendly bag, combine ingredients from chicken to fish sauce. Carefully massage the bag to dissolve the curry paste into the liquid. Squeeze out the air and seal the bag. Store in the fridge for up to 2 days or in the freezer for up to 3 months. You can also make this dish right away without marinating.

• When you are ready to cook, dump the entire bag into the pot. Try to arrange the chicken in a single layer. Make sure each piece is in contact with the liquid.

Instant Pot:

• Add everything to the Instant Pot. If it's thawed, cook for 8 minutes manual high pressure + 10 minutes for natural release. If it's frozen, cook for 15 minutes manual high pressure + 10 minutes natural release. Stir-in bamboo shoots, coconut milk cream, nut butter, and lime juice to taste. Shred or dice the chicken and add back to the pot.

Crazy Good Instant Pot Pork Carnitas

Ingredients

- Brine

- 2 Cups Orange Juice

- 4 Cups Water

- 2 Cups Apple Cider Vinegar

- 2 Bay Leaves

- ½ Cup Brown Sugar

- ½ Cup Kosher Salt

- 1 Tablespoon Cumin

- 1 Tablespoon Oregano

- 1 Tablespoon Dried Orange Peel

- 1 Tablespoon Smoked Paprika

- 1 Tablespoon Chili Powder

Pork Rub

- 3-4 Lb Pork Butt bone-in * see notes for using boneless or cubed pork shoulder

- 2 Tablespoons Cumin

- 1 Tablespoon Kosher Salt

- 1 Tablespoon Oregano

- 1½ Teaspoons Dried Orange Peel

- 2 Teaspoons Onion Powder

- 2 Teaspoons Garlic Powder

- 1 Teaspoon Ground Coriander

Cooking

- Canola Oil for Final Crisping

- ½ Cup Orange Juice

- ¼ Cup Lime Juice

- ¼ Cup Chicken Broth

Instructions

For the Brine

- Combine all brine ingredients in a large pot and stir to combine.

- Add the pork and place a lid on then stick it in the fridge for 8 hours or overnight.

For the Pork

- Remove the pork from the brine and pat dry with paper towels.

- Mix the rub together and rub all over the pork.

- Mix together the liquids and pour in the bottom of the instant pot.

- Add the pork and lid, moving the valve to seal.

- Turn to high pressure on manual and set the time for 2 hours.

- Allow a natural release for 15 minutes then turn to vent.

- Open and if the meat can be shredded remove and shred, reserving the liquid.

- If it isn't tender enough, cook for an additional 30 minutes.

- Once the meat has been shredded, heat a skillet over medium high heat with a drizzle of oil and cook the pork in batches to crisp the meat.

- Toss with a little of the juices from the instant pot and serve!

Instant Pot Mexican Stuffed Sweet Potatoes

INGREDIENTS

SWEET POTATOES

- 4 medium sweet potatoes, scrubbed
- 1½ cups water

CHICKEN

- 2 chicken breasts
- 1 10-oz. can tomatoes with green chiles, undrained, any variety
- 1 tablespoon taco seasoning

AVOCADO-JALAPEÑO SAUCE

- 1 avocado, peeled and seeded
- 1 jalapeño, stemmed
- ½ cup fresh cilantro leaves
- ½ cup water
- 2 cloves garlic
- 2 teaspoons white vinegar
- ½ teaspoon salt

QUICK GUACAMOLE

- 2 avocados
- ¼ cup avocado-jalapeño sauce
- salt

GARNISHES

- jalapeños, sliced thin
- fresh cilantro
- salsa or more tomatoes with green chiles, drained

• red onion, chopped

EQUIPMENT NEEDED

• Instant Pot

• food processor

INSTRUCTIONS

• See Notes for sweet potato and chicken cooking instructions if you do not have an Instant Pot. You can also bake your sweet potatoes in the oven while you cook the chicken in the Instant Pot to save time if you like.

• Cook your sweet potatoes: Prick sweet potatoes all over with a fork. Place steaming trivet in the bottom of Instant Pot pot then pour 1 1/2 cups water in the pot. Place sweet potatoes on trivet then secure the lid and cook on Manual, high pressure for 16 minutes. Quick release pressure and remove sweet potatoes from trivet. Set aside. Discard steaming water and rinse the cooking pot, making sure outside is very dry.

• Make your shredded chicken: combine chicken breasts, taco seasoning, and can of tomatoes with green chiles (undrained) in the pot of an Instant Pot. Do not add water. Secure lid and cook on Manual, high pressure for 20 minutes. Quick release pressure and remove chicken breasts from the pot. Shred with two forks then return to pot. Stir on Sauté mode a few minutes until sauce is absorbed.

• Meanwhile, make your sauce: combine all avocado-jalapeño sauce ingredients in the bowl of a food processor and process until smooth.

• To make guacamole, mash avocados and stir in avocado-jalapeño sauce.

• To serve: with a knife, make a slit down the top of each sweet potato and press sweet potatoes end's toward the center to push open. Top with shredded chicken, guacamole, avocado-jalapeño sauce, salsa or more tomatoes with green chiles, and garnishes. Serve immediately.

LEMON CHICKEN SOUP (INSTANT POT)

INGREDIENTS

- 2 teaspoons olive oil

- 4 medium carrots, diced

- 4 celery sticks, diced

- ½ medium onion, diced

- 4 garlic cloves, minced

- ½ teaspoon chili flakes

- 6 bone in chicken thighs

- 6 cups chicken stock

- 1 head of cauliflower, riced (about 3 cups)

- 3 large eggs

- ½ cup lemon juice

- Sea salt and pepper, to taste

- 2 ounces spinach

INSTRUCTIONS

- Turn your Instant Pot to Saute. Add the oil to the pot and add the carrots, celery, and onion and saute for 3 minutes. Add the garlic and chili flakes and cook for 1 more minute.

- Add the chicken thighs and stock to the pot. Seal the lid, turn it to Soup Mode and set the timer for 10 minutes. When the timer goes off, turn the release valve and wait until the pressure is released before opening the pot.

- While the soup is cooking, add the riced cauliflower to a pan over medium-high heat and add 1/4 cup of water. Steam until the cauliflower is soft.

- Remove the chicken thighs from the pot and shred them using 2 forks. Discard the bones.

• Whisk the eggs with the lemon juice. Slowly whisk 1 cup of the hot soup into the eggs then pour the eggs into the pot. Season to taste with sea salt and pepper.

• Return the chicken to the pot, add the cauliflower rice and the spinach, and stir.

Easy Instant Pot Ribs Recipe

Ingredients

• 2 racks pork ribs baby back or St. Louis style ribs

• Dry Rub

• 2 tablespoons chili powder

• 1 teaspoon coconut sugar (optional)

• 1 teaspoon coarse sea salt

• Sugar Free BBQ sauce optional

Instructions

• Remove membrane from back of ribs.

• Mix chili powder, salt, and coconut sugar (if using) together in a small bowl. Rub spice mixture evenly over ribs.

Instant Pot Method

• Place trivet rack in pot and add 1 cup of water. Stand the racks of ribs on the trivet.

• Cook on pressure cook high (or manual depending on which model Instant Pot you have) for 25 - 30 minutes. Allow pressure to release naturally. Finish by grilling or broiling.

INSTANT POT TACO SOUP

Equipment

• Instant Pot

Ingredients

• 1 pound Ground Beef

• ½ cup Onion

• 1 tablespoon Minced Garlic

• 1.5 tablespoons Taco Seasoning

• 1 teaspoon Kosher Salt

• 1 cup Water, divided

• 14 ounces diced tomatoes, 1 can

For Finishing

• 4 ounces Heavy Whipping Cream

• 1 cup shredded sharp cheddar cheese

• 1 Avocado, sliced (optional)

• ½ cup Green Onions, chopped (optional)

• ½ cup Cilantro, chopped

optional Non-Keto Ingredients

• Kidney Beans, cooked

• Corn, cooked

• Black Beans, cooked

Instructions

• Turn the Instant Pot to Sauté. When the indicator reads hot, add the ground beef, onions, and garlic. Break up the meat as much as possible. When the meat is no longer in a big clump, add the taco seasoning and salt, and cook for about 1 minute.

• Add ¼ cup of water and thoroughly deglaze the Instant pot liner.

• Add undrained tomatoes and remaining cup of water.

• Secure the lid on the pot. Set the Instant Pot at High pressure for 5 minutes. When cook time is complete, let pot release pressure naturally for 10 minutes, and then release all remaining pressure.

• Open the pot and stir in the whipping cream and cheese. Add more water if needed.

• Divide into four bowls, and top with sliced avocado and green onions, if using, right before serving.

Instant Pot Summer Soup

INGREDIENTS

- 1 lb. chicken breasts

- 1 28-ounce can crushed tomatoes

- 4 carrots, peeled and chopped

- 2 stalks celery, chopped

- 3 cloves minced garlic

- ½ cup farro (you can also use brown rice or small pasta)

- 6 cups chicken broth

- 2 tablespoons olive oil

- 1 teaspoon each basil and oregano

- ½ teaspoon each garlic and onion powder

- 2 teaspoons salt

- 2 zucchini, cut into small pieces

- 2–3 cups of fresh sweet corn kernels, cut off the cob

Toppings: Parmesan, lemon juice, plain yogurt, fresh herbs, freshly ground pepper, etc.

INSTRUCTIONS

- Place everything except the zucchini and sweet corn in the Instant Pot or pressure cooker. Set to high pressure for 20 minutes. Release the steam.

- Shred the chicken. Stir in the zucchini and sweet corn. Set to high pressure for another 5 minutes. Release the steam.

- Let the soup rest for a few minutes – it thickens up a bit as it cools. Season with more salt and pepper and whatever toppings you like. Aaand devour!

INSTANT POT SALSA CHICKEN

INGREDIENTS

- 4 large boneless, skinless chicken breasts, trimmed
- ¾ cup, mild or medium salsa (see notes)
- 2 T fresh-squeezed lime juice (see notes)
- salt and fresh-ground black pepper to taste for seasoning chicken
- 1 cup grated Mozzarella (or more)

INSTRUCTIONS

- Trim visible fat and undesirable parts from the chicken breasts.
- Spray the instant pot with nonstick spray, put chicken in the Instant Pot and season with salt and fresh-ground black pepper.
- Mix the salsa and fresh lime juice. (I used my fresh-frozen lime juice for this recipe.)
- Pour the salsa-lime juice mixture over the chicken.
- Lock the lid of the Instant Pot.
- Set it to MANUAL, HIGH PRESSURE, 6 minutes.
- Let pressure release naturally when the time is up, then remove the chicken breasts to a cutting board, leaving the salsa mixture in the pot.
- Turn the Instant Pot to SAUTE, HIGH TEMPERATURE, and cook until the sauce has reduced and thickened, about 8-10 minutes, but I would check it a few times.
- While the sauce cooks down, preheat oven broiler and move the rack so it's about 6 inches away from the broiler.
- Spray a baking dish with nonstick spray. Cut chicken breasts in half lengthwise and arrange them closely together in the baking dish.
- When the sauce has thickened to your linking, turn off Instant Pot and spoon the sauce over the chicken. Sprinkle with a generous amount of grated Mozzarella.

• Broil until the cheese is melted and slightly starting to brown, about 3-4 minutes, but watch it carefully if you have a powerful broiler.

• Serve hot, with diced avocado, sour cream, or Green Tabasco Sauce (affiliate link) to add at the table if desired.

INSTANT POT HUNGARIAN POT ROAST

INGREDIENTS

- 2 T olive oil, divided
- 1 beef chuck roast, about 3.5 pounds after trimming
- 2 T steak seasoning (see notes)
- 1 large onion, chopped
- 2 T sweet Hungarian paprika (or more)
- 1/2 tsp. sharp Hungarian paprika (optional, but good)
- one 12 oz. jar roasted red bell peppers, drained and chopped
- one 14.5 oz. can petite diced tomatoes, drained
- 1 cup beef broth
- fresh ground black pepper to taste (see notes)
- 1 cup sour cream

INSTRUCTIONS

- Trim fat and unwanted parts from the chuck roast; my roast was about 3.5 pounds after trimming.

- Rub the roast with steak seasoning.

- Heat 1 tablespoon olive oil in a large frying pan and brown the meat well. (I did this in a pan so I could cook onions in the Instant Pot at the same time.)

- Add the rest of the olive oil to the Instant Pot, use SAUTE, MEDIUM HEAT and brown onions.

- Add the paprika after the onions are lightly browned and cook a few minutes more.

- Then add the drained petite dice tomatoes, and one cup beef stock to the Instant Pot.

• Use a non-metal turner to scrape the bottom to be sure onions aren't stuck on, then add the browned pieces of chuck roast to the Instant Pot.

• Season with some black pepper. (The steak rub has salt so I didn't add more.)

• Set Instant Pot to MANUAL, HIGH HEAT, 40 minutes.

• When it finishes cooking, let it NATURAL RELEASE for 20 minutes, then release the rest of the pressure.

• Remove meat to a cutting board. (You might want to cover with foil to keep it warm.)

• Remove about 1/3 cup of the liquid, let it cool for a minute or two, and then whisk it into the sour cream.

• Set the Instant Pot to SAUTE, MEDIUM HEAT and start simmering to reduce the liquid in the pot. We simmered about 5 minutes.

• Drain the jar of roasted red peppers, finely chop, and add them to the Instant Pot to be part of the sauce.

• When liquid has reduced by a little less than half (or as much as you prefer), turn off Instant Pot and let the liquid cool for several minutes.

• While the sauce cools, slice meat and arrange on a serving plate.

• When sauce has slightly cooled, stir the sour cream mixture into ingredients in the Instant Pot to make the sauce. (Be sure the ingredients are not still boiling or the sour cream will separate.)

• Serve sliced meat with the sauce, either spooned over the meat or on the side. Serve hot.

INSTANT POT SOUTHWESTERN BEEF STEW

INGREDIENTS

- 2 lbs. bite-sized beef cubes, preferably chuck roast (see notes)

- 4 tsp. olive oil

- 1 medium onion, chopped small

- 1 medium Poblano chile pepper, chopped small (see notes)

- 1 T crushed or minced garlic

- 2 cans black olives, drained well and cut in half lengthwise

- 1 cup frozen cauliflower rice

- 1 14 oz. can beef broth

- 1 cup salsa (see notes)

- 1 T ground cumin

- 1 tsp. Mexican oregano

- 1 14.5 oz. can crushed tomatoes

- 2 T lime juice (see notes)

- chopped avocado, Green Tobasco Sauce, and fresh lime slices to add at the table, optional

INSTRUCTIONS

- Cut beef into bite-sized cubes. Heat a little olive oil in a big frying pan and brown the beef cubes well, seasoning with a little salt and fresh ground black pepper.

- While beef browns chop up a medium onion, a medium poblano chile, and measure out minced garlic.

- Heat 2 tsp. oil in the Instant Pot and set to SAUTE, MEDIUM HEAT. Add the chopped onion and poblano and cook 3 minutes. Then add garlic and cook one minute more.

- Drain olives and cut in half and measure out cauliflower rice.

• When beef is well-browned, add it to the Instant Pot with the onion mixture, and add the olives and cauliflower rice.

• Put beef broth, salsa, ground cumin, Mexican oregano, and crushed tomatoes into the pan you cooked the beef in. Simmer that mixture together about 5 minutes, scraping off any browned bits from the bottom. Then add that mixture to the Instant Pot.

• Set Instant Pot on MANUAL, HIGH PRESSURE, 25 minutes. When cooking time ends, let it natural release for at least 10 minutes; then release the rest of the pressure.

• Stir in lime juice, and taste to see if you want more salt.

• Serve with chopped avocado and fresh limes to add at the table if desired. This is good with Green Tabasco Sauce (affiliate link) for those who want a little more heat.

GREEN CHILE CHICKEN BURRITO BOWL

INGREDIENTS

- 4 boneless, skinless chicken breasts, trimmed and cut into strips

- 1 cup green chile salsa (see notes)

- 1 4 oz. can diced green chiles (Anaheim chiles, not jalapenos!)

- 2 avocados

- 1½ cups cherry tomatoes cut in half

- 2 green onions, thinly sliced

- 1 T olive oil

- 3 T fresh lime juice (1 T is for tossing with avocado and the rest is for the salsa. See note about the lime juice I used.)

- salt to taste

- 6 cups frozen cauliflower rice (see notes)

- 2 T olive oil

- 1 onion, chopped small

- 1 large Poblano chile pepper, seeds and stem removed and finely diced (see notes)

- 1 tsp ground cumin

- salt and fresh-ground black pepper to taste

INSTRUCTIONS

- Measure out about 6 cups frozen cauliflower rice, break apart lumps, and let it thaw on the counter.

- Trim chicken breasts and cut each one lengthwise into 2 or 3 strips (so you'll have shorter pieces of chicken when you shred the cooked chicken apart.)

- Put chicken into the Instant Pot (affiliate link) with the Salsa Verde and diced green chiles. Lock the lid and set Instant Pot to MANUAL, HIGH

PRESSURE, 8 minutes.

• When the cooking time is up, use NATURAL RELEASE for 10 minutes, then release the rest of the pressure manually.

• Remove chicken to a cutting board to cool while you turn the Instant Pot to SAUTE, MEDIUM HEAT and cook the sauce to reduce it, about 8-10 minutes.

• When it's cool, shred shred chicken apart and put it back into the Instant Pot to mix with the flavorful green chile sauce. You can use the pressure cooker to keep it warm if needed.

• While chicken cooks, dice avocados and toss with 1 T lime juice, dice tomatoes, and slice green onions. Toss the diced avocado, diced tomato, and sliced green onion with the olive oil, other 2 T fresh lime juice, and a little salt to make the salsa. (If you're doing Weekend Food Prep, I would only make half the salsa and make the rest when you eat the leftovers.)

• Chop the onion and cut out seeds and stem from the Poblano chile and finely chop the chile pepper.

• Heat 2 T olive oil in a large non-stick frying pan over medium high heat; add the chopped onion and cook 2-3 minutes. Add the finely diced poblano and cooker 2-3 minutes more. The add the ground cumin and cook about a minute more.

• Add the cauliflower rice and cook, stirring frequently, until all the liquid has evaporated, the rice is hot, and it's cooked through. This will take about 6-8 minutes, depending on how thawed the cauliflower is, but start to check after about 5 minutes.

• Season the cooked cauliflower rice with salt and fresh-ground black pepper to taste. (You can stir in some extra lime juice if you like the idea of an extra touch of lime.)

• To assemble the finished bowl meal, put a generous amount of cauliflower rice into a bowl, top with a generous scoop of the green chile chicken with sauce, and top with Tomato-Avocado salsa.

• If you're making this for Weekend Food Prep, I would only make half the amount of salsa when you eat this the first time. Refrigerate the leftover shredded chicken and cooked cauliflower rice separately. When you're ready to eat leftovers, make the rest of the salsa and heat the chicken and cauliflower rice in the microwave or in a pan on the stove.

INSTANT POT SOUTHWESTERN POT ROAST

INGREDIENTS

• 1 can (14.5 oz) reduced sodium beef broth, reduced until it's 1/2 cup strong broth

• 3 lb. beef chuck roast, visible fat trimmed and cut into several pieces (see notes)

• steak seasoning of your choice to rub on the meat (see notes)

• 2 tsp. olive oil for browning meat

• 3/4 cup + 1/2 cup low-sugar salsa (see notes)

INSTRUCTIONS

• Start reducing the can of beef broth in a pan on the stove or in the Instant Pot while you brown the meat. (We liked reducing the stock and browning the meat on the stove, but take your choice on that.)

• Trim the roast to remove visible fat (as much as you prefer),

• Heat the oil in a large frying pan and brown the meat well (or use the Instant Pot and brown it in two batches.) Put the browned beef in the Instant Pot.

• Then add the reduced beef stock to the pan and cook longer as needed until it's reduced to about 1/2 cup, scraping off the browned bits from the pan. It may or may not already be reduced that much. (If you chose to brown the meat in the Instant Pot, just reduce the stock to 1/2 cup in the saucepan and then add salsa and pour over the meat in the Instant Pot.)

• Add 3/4 cup salsa to the reduced broth and pour that cooking sauce over the meat in the Instant Pot.

• Set Instant Pot to MANUAL, HIGH PRESSURE and 35 minutes. Let the Instant Pot release pressure manually when the time is up.

• Remove the meat to a cutting board.

• We used a Fat Separator to remove some of the fat from the cooking liquid left in the Instant Pot; optional. Then add about 1/2 cup more salsa to the sauce. We used the Instant Pot to warm it while we cut the meat apart.

• Serve hot, with the sauce spooned over the meat.

INSTANT POT BALSAMIC PORK ROAST

INGREDIENTS

- 3 lb. pork loin roast
- 1 T Rosemary and Garlic Herb Rub (see notes)
- 1 T olive oil
- ¾ cup beef stock (see notes)
- ¼ cup balsamic vinegar

Direction

- Make the Rosemary and Garlic Herb Rub, if using.
- Trim unwanted fat from the pork loin roast, depending on your preference, then rub the roast on all sides with the herb rub.
- Combine 3/4 cup beef stock and 1/4 cup balsamic vinegar to make the cooking liquid.
- Turn Instant Pot to SAUTE, MEDIUM HEAT, and heat the oil.
- Then add the pork roast and brown well on all sides. Don't rush, we browned it about 3 minutes per side.
- Remove roast and use a plastic turner to scrape off any browned bits on the bottom of the pot.
- Then add the roast back into the Instant Pot and pour the cooking liquid over.
- Set Instant Pot to MANUAL, HIGH HEAT, 15 MINUTES.
- When cooking time is up, use NATURAL RELEASE to release the pressure.
- Remove the roast to a cutting board and tent with foil to keep warm.
- Set Instant Pot to SAUTE, HIGH HEAT, and simmer the cooking liquid until it's reduced as much as you prefer. (We simmered it about 10 minutes.)
- After roast rests while you reduce the sauce or at least a few minutes, slice into pieces about 1/2 inch thick.

• Serve hot with sauce to drizzle over the meat at the table.

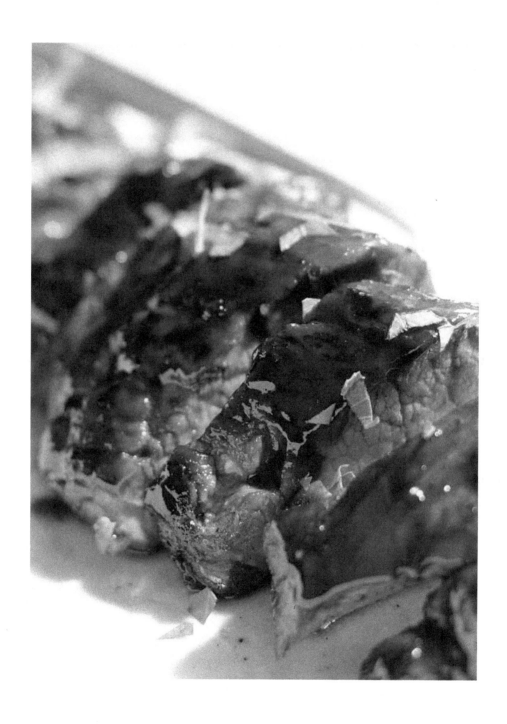

INSTANT POT CAULIFLOWER RICE GREEK CHICKEN BOWLS

INGREDIENTS

INSTANT POT INGREDIENTS:

- 4 large chicken breasts, trimmed and cut into lengthwise strips

- zest and juice of 2 lemons

- 1 T Greek Seasoning(Check ingredients for Gluten-Free)

- 2 T extra-virgin olive oil

- ¼ cup chicken stock

- ½ tsp. Greek Oregano

- ½ tsp. fresh-ground black pepper

GREEK SALSA INGREDIENTS:

- 3 medium cucumbers, chopped

- 1 cup chopped cherry tomatoes

- ¼ cup chopped Kalamata olives (or black olives)

- ¼ cup finely chopped red onion

- 4 oz. crumbled Feta Cheese

- ¼ cup Italian dressing of your choice, see notes

CAULIFLOWER RICE INGREDIENTS:

- 2 10 oz. bags frozen cauliflower rice, partly thawed (or use fresh-chopped cauliflower if you prefer)

- 1 large green bell pepper, finely chopped

- 1 small yellow onion, finely chopped

- 1 T extra-virgin olive oil

- 1 tsp. Greek Seasoning

- salt and fresh-ground black pepper to taste

INSTRUCTIONS

• Take cauliflower rice out of the freezer and let it thaw on the counter while you cook the chicken.

• Trim the chicken and cut each piece lengthwise into 2-3 strips, depending on how large the chicken breasts are. Put chicken strips into the Instant Pot.

• Grate the zest from the lemons (using a Lemon Zester is easiest). Then cut lemons in half and squeeze the juice.

• Whisk the zest and juice together with the Greek Seasoning, olive oil, chicken stock,Greek Oregano, and black pepper to make the cooking sauce. Pour the cooking sauce mixture over chicken in the Instant Pot.

• Set the Instant Pot to MANUAL, HIGH PRESSURE, 8 minutes. Then do NATURAL RELEASE for 10 minutes before you release the rest of the pressure.

• When the pressure has all been released, use a slotted spoon to remove chicken to a cutting board, leaving the flavorful sauce in the Instant Pot. (If it seems like there's too much liquid in the Instant Pot, cook on SAUTE / HIGH HEAT for a few minutes to reduce the liquid.) Shred chicken apart with two forks, put it back in the Instant Pot, and stir gently so the chicken is coated with liquid. Keep chicken warm on the low setting while you prep the other ingredients.

• To make Greek Salsa, chop the cucumbers, tomatoes, Kalamata olives (or black olives), and red onion. Put those chopped ingredients in a bowl, stir in the 1/4 cup Italian dressing, and then gently stir in the crumbled Feta.

• Chop the yellow onion and green pepper.

• If you're using fresh cauliflower, trim the cauliflower and discard the leaves. To use a food processor to chop up the cauliflower into "rice," first cut the cauliflower (including the stems) into small pieces. Then pulse the cauliflower pieces using the steel blade in the food processor until it's finely chopped. (This recipe has good photos and instructions for doing that.) You can also make the "rice" by grating larger pieces of cauliflower with a large standing box grater.

• Heat the tablespoon of olive oil in a large non-stick pan over medium-high heat, add the green pepper and onion, and cook about 3 minutes or until the vegetables are softened and starting to brown.

• Add the Greek seasoning and cook 1 minute more; then add the chopped semi-thawed frozen cauliflower (or fresh cauliflower) and cook, turning a few times, until the cauliflower is heated through and some liquid has evaporated, about 3-4 minutes. (Taste cauliflower to see when it's hot and cooked through; fresh cauliflower will take a bit longer to cook.) Season the cauliflower rice with salt and fresh-ground black pepper.

• To assemble the bowl, put some of the hot cauliflower rice in the bottom of a serving bowl. On top of the rice put a generous scoop of the shredded lemon chicken from the slow cooker, and then top that with a scoop of the Greek salsa mixture. Serve right away.

• You can keep the shredded lemon chicken in the fridge for a day or two and reheat in a pan or in the microwave. For the Cauliflower Rice and the Greek salsa mixture, I would make that fresh each time when you're eating the leftovers.

SPICY SHREDDED CHICKEN LETTUCE WRAP TACOS

INGREDIENTS

SPICY CHICKEN TACOS:

• 4 boneless, skinless chicken breasts, trimmed and cut into strips lengthwise (see notes)

• 1 cup mild or medium low-sugar tomato salsa (see notes)

• ¼ cup chicken stock (omit for slow cooker version)

• 1 7 oz. can diced green chiles, not drained (see notes)

• 1 T Cholula hot sauce, or other Mexican hot sauce of your choice (see notes)

• 2 T fresh-squeezed lime juice (see notes)

• 1 tsp. onion powder

• 2 heads iceberg lettuce, washed if needed

AVOCADO SALSA:

• 2 medium avocados, diced into small pieces

• ¾ cup chopped fresh cilantro (more or less to taste)

• ¼ cup chopped red onion

• ¼ cup fresh-squeezed lime juice (or maybe a bit less if you're not a big fan of lime)

INSTRUCTIONS

INSTANT POT INSTRUCTIONS:

• Trim visible fat and other unwanted parts from chicken breasts and cut each one into three or four strips lengthwise. Spray the inside of the Instant Pot with olive oil or non-stick spray and arrange the chicken strips in the pot.

• Combine the salsa, chicken stock, diced green chiles, onion powder, hot sauce, lime juice, and onion powder to make the spicy sauce. Pour over the chicken in the Instant Pot.

• Lock the lid, set the Instant Pot to MANUAL, HIGH PRESSURE, 8 minutes.

• When the 8 minutes cooking time has finished, let the Instant Pot NATURAL RELEASE for 10 minutes, then turn the valve to quick release the rest of the pressure.

• Remove the chicken strips to a cutting board to cool. Turn the Instant Pot to SAUTE/LOW HEAT and let the liquid simmer until it's cooked down to about 1/2 cup. (This takes about 5-10 minutes.) While the liquid reduces, use two forks to shred chicken apart.

• Peel and dice the avocados and toss with the lime juice (in a bowl that's big enough for all the salsa ingredients.) Add the chopped cilantro and chopped red onion and stir gently to combine.

• Cut iceberg lettuce heads in half and wash in salad spinner if needed. Peel off two pieces of lettuce to make a "cup" and fill with a scoop of chicken mixture and a scoop of avocado salsa. Eat tacos with your hands.

CPSIA information can be obtained
at www.ICGtesting.com
Printed in the USA
LVHW100724160621
690353LV00019B/1726